Quinoa Recipe Cookbook

One stop shop for all Quinoa recipe needs

AMARPREET SINGH

Publisher - The Thought Flame

THE THOUGHT FLAME
TURNING SPARK INTO FLAME

info@thethoughtflame.com

www.thethoughtflame.com

Table of Contents

Introduction 1

5 Health Benefits of Quinoa That May

Surprise You 3

Conclusion 83

About Us 84

Author 86

Introduction

For many years quinoa has been growing in popularity and is considered one of the best super foods on the market today. What is it about this grain that has health experts excited and that has many people looking for recipes to include this ingredient?

There are many reasons as to why you should begin using quinoa in your diet on a daily basis and many delicious recipes that you can find that include this healthy grain. In this eBook you will only find recipes that include this ingredient and that will help you live a healthier life style in the long run.

With quinoa you will be able to make recipes that only take a few minutes and that will leave you feeling full throughout the day. So, what are you waiting for? Let's get started with some healthy quinoa recipes and learn what it is exactly that makes this grain one of the best grains that you can consume.

5 Health Benefits of Quinoa That May Surprise You

It is no secret that quinoa is a grain that is growing in popularity as the years pass. It is so popular in fact that it is considered one of the world's most popular "superfoods" available today. Quinoa is not only loaded with a ton of protein, but it is loaded with fiber and important minerals that you need.

There are many health benefits to including quinoa in your diet today and many of these benefits may surprise you.

1. It is Incredibly Nutritious

Quinoa is one of the most popular grains used today because of the fact that it is incredibly nutritious. While many people may automatically assume that this grain is a cereal grain (since it looks very similar to many cereal grains), that is not the case. In fact quinoa is a pseudocerael. What does this mean? All it means is that quinoa is a seed and that is made and eaten in a way that is similar to any other grain out there.

What is more surprising is how long quinoa has been around. Research has shown us that quinoa has been around as early as the Incan Empire where the Inca's referred to this grain as the mother of all grains. It was so popular back then that many Inca's swore that this grain was sacred.

Over thousands of years this superfood has been consumed by thousands and the popularity of this super food continues to grow to this very day. There are many products all over the world that contain this ingredient especially any restaurant or super market that sells natural foods.

There are exactly 3 types of quinoa available today: red quinoa, black quinoa and white quinoa. To get an idea of how healthy and nutritious this food staple is for you, here is a breakdown of what 1 cup of cooked quinoa contains:

-8 Grams of Protein

-5 Grams of Fiber

-58% of Manganese

-30% of Magnesium

-28% of Phosphorus

-19% of Folate

-18% of Copper

-15% of Iron

-13% of Zinc

-9% of Potassium

-Over 10% of Vitamin B6, B1 and B2

-Small Amounts of Vitamin E, Calcium and B3

In 1 cup of cooked quinoa there are only 226 calories, 39 grams of carbohydrates and only 4 grams of fat. You will not find any other grain that is as nutritious as quinoa.

2. Contains Quercetin and Kaempferol

While you are looking for the health benefits of many real and nutritious foods, there are foods that you will want to find that go above the call of supplying healthy vitamins and minerals that we all need.

In quinoa there are many trace nutrients you will find and some of the nutrients that you will find are extremely healthy. The two nutrients that you will find in quinoa are two flavonoids known as Kaempferol and Quercetin. These two nutrients are antioxidants which have shown to help improve the overall health of your body in the long run. They help to relive inflammation, viruses, potential cancer and depression effects within your body.

When your add quinoa to your diet on a regular basis, you will help to increase the amount of antioxidants you take in and will help to improve your health in the long run.

3. Quinoa Is Very High In Fiber

There is no other grain available today that contains as much fiber as quinoa does. On average quinoa contains about 17 to 27 grams of quinoa per cooked cup. This is extremely high especially when you compare it to other grains that are available.

The downside to this fiber is that it is considered to be insoluble fiber, which is not as helpful as soluble fiber, but hey! It is still fiber in our book. This fiber has been proven to help reduce the chance of having high blood sugar, high cholesterol and high body fat.

4. It is Gluten Free

Today many people unfortunately are gluten intolerant and as such it can be hard to find recipes and dishes that do not contain gluten. For people who suffer from gluten intolerance, they will find quinoa to be their saving grace. Quinoa is the perfect ingredient to use in virtually any kind of recipe, especially if the person in question is having a problem giving up foods such as pasta and bread.

There have been many studies conducted that have shown when you use quinoa in a dish instead of typical gluten packed ingredients, it can help increase how nutritious and antioxidant rich your dish becomes. Quinoa is something I definitely recommend for people who have an aversion to gluten products as this ingredients will allow you to enjoy classic dishes without gluten.

5. Quinoa Is Packed Full of Protein

If you are looking for a type of food that is extremely high in protein, quinoa is the food you have been looking for. The important thing to remember here is that protein is simply made out of various amino acids. Some foods out there today simply do not contain all of the amino acids that you need in order to make a complete protein.

However, that is where quinoa can come into the picture. Quinoa is the exception to many grains out there as it contains all of the amino acids needed to make a complete protein and because of this it is considered to be one of the best sources of protein than any other grain available today.

There are many reasons to use quinoa is most of the dishes you prepare such as that it is packed full of protein that you need to it is one of the most nutritious food staples that you will find today. When you use quinoa in many dishes today, your possibilities to make great tasting food is endless. This eBook is solely dedicated to this superfood and in this eBook you will find the most nutritious and great tasting recipes that you will find anywhere.

Traditional Quinoa Tabbouleh

This dish is not only high in fiber, but is packed with high quality protein as well. This recipe will help you to make a dish that is similar to rice, but that has a much milder flavor.

Total Prep Time: 30 Minutes

Serves: 2

Ingredients:

-1 ¾ Cup of Water, Warm

-1 Cup of Quinoa, Uncooked

-¼ Cup of Cucumber, Finely Chopped

-½ Cup of Tomato, Seeded and Chopped Coarsely

-¼ Cup of Raisins, Your Favorite Brand

-½ Cup of Parsley, Fresh and Chopped Finely

-¼ of Lemon Juice, Fresh

-2 tsp. of Onion, Fresh and Minced

-2 Tbsp. of Onions, Fresh, Green and Chopped Finely

-1 Tbsp. of Olive Oil, Extra Virgin Preferable

-Dash of Salt and Black Pepper For Taste

Directions:

1. In a medium sized saucepan bring your water and uncooked quinoa together. Stir and then bring to a boil. Cover and continue to cook until all of the water has been absorbed at a simmering heat.

2. Remove pan from heat and fluff your quinoa with a fork. Add in your remaining ingredients and stir to thoroughly combine everything. Cover and allow to stand for at least 1 minute. Serve while it is at room temperature.

Beet and Kumquat Quinoa Salad

This filling and hearty salad features beets, kumquats, blood oranges and avocado, giving this dish some vibrant color. It is packed full of nutrients and vitamins that will help you feel much healthier in the long run

Total Prep Time: 25 Minutes

Serves: 2

Ingredients For The Salad:

-1 Cup of Quinoa, Uncooked

-1 ¾ Cup of Water

-1 Cup of Avocado, Peeled and Diced Finely

-½ tsp. of Salt, Divided Evenly

-1 Cup of Blood Orange Sections, Chopped Into Small Pieces

-6 Kumquats, Whole, Seeded and Sliced Into Small Pieces

-2 Beets, Medium In Size, Cooked and Cut Into Small Wedges

Ingredients For The Dressing:

-¼ tsp. of Salt

-¼ Cup of Onions, Green and Chopped Finely

-2 Tbsp. of Blood Orange, Juice

-1 Tsp. of Lemon Rind, Finely Grated

-1 Tbsp. of Lemon Juice, Fresh

-2 tsp. of Cilantro, Chopped Finely

-¼ tsp. of Paprika

-¼ tsp. of Coriander, Ground

-¼ tsp. of Cumin, Ground

-3 Tbsp. of Olive Oil, Extra Virgin

Directions:

1. Prepare your dressing first. To do this combine all of your ingredients into a medium sized mixing bowl and stir with a whisk to thoroughly combine. Set the bowl aside.

2. Next take your quinoa and water and combine them together in a small sized pot. Bring to a boil and then reduce the heat to simmer. Allow quinoa to simmer for 20 minutes or until all of the water has been absorbed. Remove from heat and fluff with a fork.

3. Next using a medium sized mixing bowl combine the rest of your ingredients with your quinoa and toss gently until all of the

ingredients are mixed well. Serve into small sized salad bowls and top with dressing.

Red Pepper and Quinoa Chili

If you are looking for the perfect dish to warm you up on a cold winter's night, this is the recipe for you. This recipe makes a chili that is packed full of nutritious vegetables and quinoa that will certainly leave you feeling warm afterwards.

Total Prep Time: 25 minutes

Serves: 4

Ingredients:

-2 Red Bell Peppers, Chopped Finely

-2 Pablano Chili Peppers, Chopped Finely

-4 tsp. of Olive Oil

-3 Cups of Zucchini, Chopped Into Small Pieces

-1 ½ Cup of Onion, Chopped Finely

-4 Cloves of Garlic, Fresh and Minced

-1 tsp. of Cumin, Ground

-1 Tbsp. of Chili Powder, Ground

-½ Cup of Water, Warm

-½ tsp. of Paprika, Spanish Style and Smoked

-¼ tsp. of Salt

-1/3 Cup of Quinoa, Rinsed and Uncooked

-1, 14.5 Ounce Can of Tomatoes With Chipotles, Fire Roasted and Diced

-1, 15 Ounce Can of Pinto Beans, Rinsed and Drained

-1 Cup of Vegetable Juice, Low Sodium

Directions:

1. Preheat your broiler.

2. While your broiler heats up prepare all of

your ingredients by chopping, rinsing, draining or mincing them. Then using a medium sized sauté pan, add in your olive oil and sauté your chopped zucchini, garlic and onions for about 4 minutes or until your onions become translucent. Then add in your spices. Stir to combine.

3. Next add in your pepper and chilies into your saucepan along with your warm water. Stir to combine your ingredients and bring to a rolling boil. Add in your remaining ingredients and stir thoroughly to combine.

4. Reduce your heat to low and cover. Allow your mixture to simmer for 20 minutes or until your quinoa becomes tender. Remove and serve while piping hot.

Classic Bajane Alla Chickpea

The term Bajane comes from a term in Provence that is translated as the midday meal. In Provence Chickpeas are food staples and just like with this recipe, the locals there know exactly how to create an excellent dish using this tasty ingredient.

Total Prep Time: 25 Minutes

Serves: 4

Ingredients To Prepare Quinoa:

-1 Clove of Garlic, Fresh and Minced

-2 tsp. of Olive Oil, Extra Virgin

-1 Cup of Vegetable Broth, Organic Preferable

-1 Cup of Water, Warm

-1 Cup of Uncooked Quinoa

-1 ½ tsp. of Thyme, Fresh and Finely Chopped

-¼ tsp. of Salt

Ingredients For Your Chickpea Mixture:

-2 tsp. of Olive Oil, Extra Virgin and Divided Equally

-2 Cups of Leeks, Thinly Sliced

-4 Garlic Cloves, Chopped

-2 ½ Cups of Fennel Bulb, Sliced Finely

-1 ¾ Cups of Carrots, Sliced Thinly

-½ Cup of White Wine, Your Choice

-½ tsp. of Fennel Seeds, Fresh

-4 tsp. of Thyme, Fresh, Chopped Finely and Divided Equally

-1 Cup of Vegetable Broth, Organic

-Dash of Salt and Pepper For Taste

-1 Tbsp. of Lemon Juice, Fresh

-1 Package of Baby Spinach, Fresh

Directions:

1. To prepare your quinoa, heat up your olive oil in a medium sized saucepan over medium to high heat. Saute your garlic for about 1 minute. Then add in your broth and the remaining ingredients. Stir to combine and reduce the heat. Allow to simmer until all of the liquid has been absorbed. Fluff your quinoa with a fork. Remove from heat and set aside.

2. To prepare your chickpea mixture, sauté your garlic cloves, fennel bulbs, carrots and fennel seeds together until all of the vegetables are nice and tender. Then add in your wine and allow to cook until the liquid completely evaporates.

3. Next stir in your broth, chickpeas and thyme and allow to cook until all of the ingredients are

completely heated through. Remove your pan from heat and add in your remaining ingredients.

4. Stir to combine all of your ingredients and then spoon the mixture into 4 separate bowls. Top with your cooked quinoa and serve with ½ tsp. of Thyme used as garnish. Enjoy.

Delicious Quinoa Salad With Parsley and Artichoke

This dish, while it cleverly fools the eye, is the perfect addition to any Passover dinner table. While many think quinoa is a grain, it is in fact a seed, allowing you to enjoy this dish during one of the most important holidays of the year.

Total Prep Time: 30 Minutes

Serves: 8

Ingredients:

-1 Tbsp. of Olive Oil

-½ tsp. of Thyme, Fresh and Finely Chopped

-1 Cup of Onions, Sweet and Chopped Finely

-1 Cup of Chicken Broth, Low Sodium and Fat Free

-1 Package of Artichoke Hearts, Frozen and Thawed

-½ Cup of Quinoa, Fully Cooked

-5 tsp. of Lemon Rind, Fresh and Grated

-1 Cup of Parsley, Freshly Chopped

-1 ½ Tbsp. of Lemon Juice

-¼ tsp. of Salt, Kosher For Taste

Directions:

1. Using a medium sized saucepan, sauté your onion and thyme over medium to high heat until your onions are tender and translucent.

2. Next add in your artichokes and sauté for just 2 more minutes. Then add in your quinoa and brother. Reduce the heat and bring your mixture to a simmer.

3. Cover your mixture and allow to cook for 18 minutes or until the liquid is completely absorbed. Remove from heat.

4. Next add in your salt, parsley, rind and juice and stir until all of the ingredients are thoroughly combined. Serve while the mixture is still warm.

Dried Pistachios, Cherries and Quinoa

This dish makes an excellent side dish to compliment virtually any meal. Feel free to serve this completely chilled or room temperature.

Total Prep Time: 20 Minutes

Serves: 3

Ingredients:

-1/3 Cup of White Wine, Dry

-1 ¾ Cups of Quinoa, Uncooked

-3 Tbsp. of Shallots, Finely Chopped

-2 Tbsp. + 2 tsp. of Olive Oil, Extra Virgin

-2 Cups of Water

-½ tsp. of Salt

-3 Tbsp. of Lemon Juice, Fresh

-¼ tsp. of Black Pepper, Ground

-½ Cup of Sweet Cherries, Dried and Finely Chopped

-½ Cup of Pistachios, Dry Roasted and Finely Chopped

-¼ Cup of Parsley, Fresh and Finely Chopped

-¼ Cup of Mint, Fresh and Finely Chopped

Directions:

1. Completely rinse and drain your uncooked quinoa. Afterwards while using a large sized saucepan sitting over medium to high heat, sauté your shallots for about 2 minutes or until they become tender. Then add in your water, wine and salt to your pan. Increase the heat and bring your mixture to a rolling boil.

2. Add your quinoa to your pan and cover. Reduce the heat to a simmer and allow the quinoa to cook for about 15 minutes or until the liquid is completely absorbed. Fluff your quinoa with a fork and set aside to use later.

3. In a large mixing bowl combine your pepper, 2 Tbsp. of olive oil and lemon juice. Stir your ingredients together using a whisk until thoroughly blended. Then add in your quinoa

and remaining ingredients to the bowl and gently toss until of the ingredients are mixed well. Serve and enjoy.

Fresh Parsley and Quinoa Salad

If you have ever wanted to enjoy a vibrant colored salad, this is certainly the dish for you. Featuring fresh parsley and dried apricots, this dish not only looks good, but tastes great as well.

Total Prep Time: 25 Minutes

Serves: 2

Ingredients:

-½ Cup of Quinoa, Uncooked

-1 Cup of Water

-½ Cup of Celery, Sliced Thinly

-¾ Cup of Parsley Leaves, Fresh

-½ Cup of Green Onion, Sliced Thinly

-½ Cup of Dried Apricots, Chopped Finely

-3 Tbsp. of Lemon Juice, Fresh

-1 Tbsp. of Olive Oil

-1 Tbsp. of Honey

-Dash of Salt and Pepper For Taste

-¼ Cup of Pumpkinseed Kernels, Unsalted and Toasted

Directions:

1. In a medium sized saucepan, bring both your quinoa and water together until the mixture reaches a rolling boil. Cover with a lid and reduce the heat. Allow your quinoa to simmer for 20 minutes or until all of the water has been completely absorbed. Fluff your quinoa with a fork.

2. Then add in your dried apricots, parsley, onions and celery and stir until your ingredients are mixed well.

3. In a small bowl whisk together your salt, pepper, lemon juice, olive oil and honey until the mixture is completely smooth. Then add this mixture into your quinoa mixture and toss until everything is mixed well. Top with your pumpkinseed kernels and serve immediately.

Savory Curried Quinoa Salad

Inspired by classic Indian dishes, this quinoa rich recipe is one of the easiest quinoa recipes that you can find. The curry powder that you use helps to spice things up, making this a dish that you will love to enjoy especially when you are craving something spicy.

Total Prep Time: 25 Minutes

Serves: 6

Ingredients:

-2 tsp. of Curry Powder, Madras Brand Preferable

-1 tsp. of Olive Oil

-2 Cup of Water, Warm

-1 Clove of Garlic, Crushed

-1 Cup of Quinoa, Uncooked

-3/4 tsp. of Salt, Kosher

-1/2 Cup of Celery, Diced Finely

-1 Ripe Mango, Peeled and Diced Into Small Pieces

-1/4 Cup of Green Onions, Sliced Thinly

-3 Tbsp. of Currants

-3 Tbsp. of Cilantro, Fresh and Finely Chopped

-2 tsp. of Mint, Fresh and Finely Chopped

-¼ Cup of Cucumber, Peeled and Diced Finely

-1, 6 Ounce Carton of Yogurt, Plain and Low-Fat

-1, 5 Ounce Package of Baby Spinach, Fresh

Directions:

1. In a medium sized saucepan over medium to high heat up your olive oil. Next add in your garlic and curry and cook for at least 2 minute. Then add in your quinoa and 2 cups of water to your pan and bring to a boil. Cover with a lid and reduce the heat. Allow your quinoa to simmer for 16 minutes or until the liquid has been completely absorbed. Remove from heat, add in your salt and fluff your quinoa with a fork. Allow to cool completely.

2. Next add in your green onions, cilantro, mango, celery and currants to your cooled

quinoa. Toss gently until everything is mixed thoroughly.

3. In a small bowl combine your yogurt, cucumber and mint together and stir well.

4. Divide up your spinach among 6 different plates and top with at least ¾ to 1 cup of your quinoa mixture and 2 Tbsp. of your mango mix. Serve and enjoy.

Shitake Mushrooms with Leeks and Quinoa

Since quinoa is known as a popular super food in today's world, there are now an endless amount of recipes including this ingredient. One such delicious recipe is this one and this dish has an excellent aroma that will leave your mouth watering.

Total Prep Time: 22 Minutes

Serves: 4

Ingredients:

-1 Cup of Water, Warm

-2 Cups of Vegetable Broth, Fat Free and Low Sodium

-1 ½ Cups of Quinoa, Uncooked and Thoroughly Rinsed

-Dash of Salt and Pepper For Taste

-1 Tbsp. of Olive Oil, Divided Evenly

-3 Tbsp. of Parsley, Fresh and Chopped Finely

-3 Cups of Leeks, Sliced Thinly

-4 Cups of Shitake Mushrooms, Just The Caps and Thinly Sliced

-¼ Cup of White Wine, Dry

-½ Cup of Walnuts, Chopped Coarsely

-1 ½ Cups of Red Bell Pepper, Chopped Finely

Directions:

1. Combine your salt, water and broth together in a large sized saucepan and bring to a nice rolling boil. Then stir in your quinoa, reduce the heat and cover. Allow your quinoa to cook for 15 minutes or until the liquid has been fully absorbed. Fluff with a fork and remove from heat.

2. Next add in your parsley, oil and black pepper to your cooked quinoa and stir until everything is mixed well. Set aside.

3. Using a medium size non-stick skillet, heat up your remaining oil and sauté your leeks for about 6 minutes or until they have been completely wilted. Then add in your mushroom caps, wine and bell pepper and cook until they have become tender. Season with some salt and pepper and remove from heat.

4. Serve 1 Cup of quinoa into serving bowls and top with 1 ¼ Cup of your vegetable mixture. Top with your walnuts and serve when ready.

Filling Black Bean and Quinoa Salad

If you are looking for a dish that will really impress your guests at dinner, this is certainly the dish for you. Served on a bed of baby spinach, this dish is both colorful and great tasting

Total Prep Time: 30 Minutes

Serves: 5

Ingredients:

-1 ½ Cups of Quinoa, Uncooked

-3 Tbsp. of Olive Oil, Divided

-3 Cups of Vegetable Broth, Organic

-1, 14 Ounce Pack of Tofu, Reduced Fat and Cut Into Small Cubes

-1 1/4 tsp. of Salt, Evenly Divided

-1 Cup of Basil, Freshly Chopped

-3 Tbsp. of Lemon Juice, Fresh

-2 Tbsp. of Dijon Mustard

-2 tsp. of Lemon Rind, Grated

-1 tsp. of Sugar

-1/2 tsp. of Black Pepper, Ground

-3 Cloves of Garlic, Minced

-4 Cups of Tomato, Finely Chopped

-1, 10 Ounce Pack of Lima Beans, Frozen

-1/2 Cup of Green Onions, Thinly Sliced

-1/2 Cup of Carrots, Chopped

-1, 15 Ounce Can of Black Beans, Drained and Rinsed

Directions:

1. Combine both your vegetable broth and quinoa together in a medium sized saucepan. Bring this to a boil over medium to high heat. Cover with a lid and reduce the heat. Allow your quinoa mixture to simmer for 15 minutes or until all of the liquid is has been absorbed. Remove from heat.

2. Place your tofu on a couple of layers of paper towels and cover with some more paper towels. Leave your tofu to stand for 5 minutes.

3. Then in using a medium sized non-stick skillet over medium to high heat, add in your olive oil and add your tofu into it. Season with some salt and sauté tofu for 9 minutes or until it becomes lightly brown. Remove from heat and allow to cool completely.

4. In a medium sized mixing bowl combine your 2 Tbsp. of Oil, Salt, basil, lemon juice, sugar, Dijon mustard, lemon rind and pepper together. Whisk together until everything is thoroughly blended.

5. Stir in your quinoa and toss until mixed thoroughly together.

6. Lastly cook your lima beans exactly as the package directs and then allow to cool completely before adding that and the rest of your ingredients to your quinoa mixture. Toss to combine thoroughly. Pour onto a bed of fresh baby spinach and serve immediately.

Stuffed Squash

As we creep closer to Thanksgiving, it seems the only thing that we seem to crave all of the time is Pumpkin. Well with this recipe you will get the chance to nip your craving in the butt as well as have the chance to store some extra for later.

Total Prep Time: 50 Minutes

Serves: 4

Ingredients:

-4 Squashes, Golden Nugget Variety

-Some Cooking Spray

-½ Cup of Carrot, Chopped Finely

-½ Cup of Onion, Chopped Finely

-½ Cup of Water, Warm

-2 Cloves of Garlic, Minced

-2 Cups of Quinoa, Fully Cooked

-2 Tbsp. of Parsley, Fresh and Finely Chopped

-½ tsp. of Thyme, Fresh and Finely Chopped

-Dash of Salt and Pepper For Taste

-¾ Cup of Monterey Jack Cheese, Shredded and 2% (Divide Evenly)

-2 Links of Turkey Sausage, Italian Style and With The Casings Removed

Directions:

1. To prepare your squash you will want to cut the top quarter of each squash. Make sure that you save the tops and remove all of the seeds from the inside of each squash. Place your squash into a small microwave safe baking dish and fill the baking dish up with at least 1 inch of water. Place the dish into your microwave and microwave on high for 15 minutes. Remove from your microwave and allow to cool completely.

2. Next preheat your oven to 350 degrees. While your oven preheats heat up a large sized skillet over medium to high heat. Make sure that you coat your skillet with a generous amount of cooking spray and add in your

sausage. Sauté for at least 5 minutes or until the sausage is browned completely.

3. Remove your sausage and then ad in your garlic, carrots and onions to your pan and sauté for about 2 minutes, making sure to stir frequently. Then add in your water and allow it to come to a boil. Reduce your heat to medium heat and then cook for an additional 8 minutes or until your carrots until it is tender.

4. In a large sized mixing bowl combine your quinoa, sausage, parsley, salt, pepper, carrot mixture and thyme together. Then add in your cheese and stir until all of the ingredients are mixed well.

5. Stuff your squash with your quinoa mixture and top with 1 heaping Tbsp. of Cheese. Place your stuffed squash into a baking dish and place your squash tops into your dish. Bake at 350 degrees for at least 20 minutes or until the squash are thoroughly heated through.

6. Place your broiler on high and broil your squash for 4 minutes or until the cheese turns gold in color. Remove from oven and serve immediately.

Easy Quinoa Grecian Salad

Once you discover quinoa and realize that it has the potential to make a lot of recipes that are absolutely delicious, it is an ingredient that you will want to use in all of your recipes. This recipe tastes great and allows you to make a dish that is extremely colorful

Total Prep Time: 25 Minutes

Serves: 5

Ingredients:

-2 cups of Quinoa, Uncooked

-2 Tbsp. of Olive Oil, Extra Virgin

-3 Cups of Chicken Broth, Low Sodium and Fat Free

-1 tsp. of Mint, Fresh and Minced

-1 tsp. of Lemon Rind, Grated

-2 tsp. of Lemon Juice, Fresh

-1 tsp. of Vinegar, Sherry

-½ tsp. of Sea Salt

-1 Cup of Radicchio, Sliced Thinly

-1 Cup of Tomatoes, Cherry and Sliced Into Thin Quarters

-½ Cup of Cucumber, Chopped Into Small Pieces

-½ Cup of Yellow Pepper, Chopped Into Small Pieces

-3 Tbsp. of Kalamata Olives, Pitted and Chopped Finely

-1 Tbsp. of Shallots, Minced

-1/3 Cup of Feta Cheese, Low Fat and Crumbled

Directions:

1. Take your uncooked quinoa and put into a small bowl. Cover your quinoa with some water and allow to stand for about 5 minutes. After 5 minutes Rinse your quinoa and drain.

2. While your quinoa sits fill up a medium sized soup pot with your water and bring to a rolling boil. Pour your quinoa into the pot and cover with a lid. Reduce your heat and allow the quinoa to simmer for at least 15 minutes or until all of the liquid had been absorbed. Uncover and fluff your cooked quinoa with a fork. Remove from heat and allow to cool.

3. In a medium sized mixing bowl combine your sherry vinegar, olive oil, lemon rind, sea salt, mint and lemon juice together until all of

the ingredients are mix well. Add in your cooked quinoa and the remaining ingredients and toss to combine. Serve while at room temperature and enjoy.

Savory Sake Salmon and Quinoa

Who doesn't enjoy a little sake? With Sake's slightly nutty flavor, it is able to compliment the quinoa used in this dish to make a truly delicious meal that will surely impress your entire family.

Total Prep Time: 3 Hours and 40 Minutes

Serves: 4

Ingredients:

-1 Pound of Salmon, Sliced Into Fillets

-2 tsp. of Sugar, Divided Evenly

-1 ½ Cups of Sake, Evenly Divided

-1 tsp. of Salt

-½ tsp. of Chili Paste

-2 Cloves of Garlic, Minced

-1 tsp. of Butter, Slightly Melted

-1 Cup of Quinoa, uncooked

-1 ½ tsp. of Olive Oil, Extra Virgin and Evenly Divided

-½ Cup of Red Bell Pepper, Chopped Finely

-½ Cup of Carrot, Finely Chopped

-¼ Cup of Onion, Finely Chopped

-1 Cup of Water, Warm

-½ Cup of Orange Juice, Fresh Preferably

-¼ tsp. of Salt

-1 Tbsp. of Parsley, Fresh and Chopped Finely

Directions:

1. With the skin placed with the skin side down, season your salmon with 1 tsp. of Sugar and 1 tsp. of Salt. Cover your newly seasoned salmon with some plastic wrap and place in your fridge to chill for the next 2 hours.

2. After 2 hours take out your seasoned salon and rinse under some cold water. Pat the salmon down with a paper towel to dry. In a small mixing bowl combine your sake, chili paste, 1 tsp. of Sugar and garlic. Pour into a Ziploc bag and add in your salmon, seal your bag and allow your salmon to marinate in your fridge for 1 hour, making sure that you turn your salmon every once in a while.

3. While your salmon marinates rinse your quinoa with some water and drain. Then melt your butter in a medium sized saucepan over some medium heat. Add in your olive oil and then sauté your onions, peppers and carrots for

about 2 minutes or until your onions become tender. Then add in your quinoa and quickly add in your water, ½ cup of your sake, some extra salt and orange juice. Allow to cook until mixture comes to a rolling boil. Cover with a lid and reduce your heat so the mixture can simmer for at least 20 minutes or until the liquid has been fully absorbed. Remove from heat and then fluff your quinoa with a fork.

4. Next preheat your oven to 450 degrees. While your oven preheats remove your marinating salmon and remove your salmon from the bag. Hold on to the marinade and pour into a small sized saucepan and heat up over medium to high heat. You will want to cook marinade until there is only about 2 Tbsp. of the marinade left.

5. Place your salmon onto a baking pan and brush with some olive oil. Make sure your place the salmon with the skin side up. Place into

your oven and cook for about 3 minutes or until it turns a nice golden brown in color. Turn the salmon over and continue to cook for an additional 5 minutes. Remove from oven and serve the salmon immediately with your quinoa. Enjoy.

Roasted Garlic and Spinach With Quinoa

With this savory dish you will be able to enjoy a dish that is not only very filling, but that will have a nice crunch as well. It is another great and colorful dish that will lighten up your dinner table.

Total Prep Time: 1 Hour and 25 Minutes

Serves: 4

Ingredients:

-1 Garlic, The Whole Head

-1 Tbsp. of Olive Oil

-1 Tbsp. of Shallots, Chopped Finely

-¼ tsp. of Red Pepper, Crushed

-½ Cup of Quinoa, Uncooked, Rinsed and Drained

-1 Tbsp. of White Wine, Dry

-1 Cup of Chicken Broth, Low Sodium and Fat Free

-½ Cup of Baby Spinach, Whole Leaves

-1/3 Cup of Tomato, Seeded and Finely Chopped

-1 Tbsp. of Parmesan Cheese, Fresh and Shaved

-¼ tsp. of Salt

Directions:

1. Preheat your oven to 350 degrees.

2. While your oven heats up prepare your head

of garlic by separating it into whole cloves. You will then need to wrap the head of garlic in aluminum foil while reserving the remaining garlic to use for later. Place your wrapped head of garlic into your oven and allow to bake for 1 hour. Remove from oven after 1 hour and allow to cool for about 10 minutes.

3. Once cooled squeeze your garlic to extract the garlic pulp and throw away the skin of the garlic.

4. Using a medium sized saucepan, heat some oil in it over medium to high heat. Add in your shallots and red pepper and cook for about 1 minute. Next add in your quinoa and cook for an additional 2 minutes, making sure to stir your mixture constantly. Then add in your white win and allow the quinoa to cook until the liquid has been fully absorbed.

5. Next add in your chicken broth and allow your mixture to come to boil. Reduce your heat

and allow your mixture to simmer for about 15 minutes or until the liquid has been fully absorbed. Remove from heat and use a fork to fluff your quinoa.

6. Then stir in you spinach, cheese, salt, tomato and garlic pulp until all of the ingredients are thoroughly mixed. Serve immediately.

Delicious Quinoa Salad with Pistachios and Apricots

There is nothing healthier than enjoying a quinoa salad for either lunch or dinner. With this dish you will be able to just that while enjoying a dish that will help get you through your busy day

Total Prep Time: 30 Minutes

Serves: 4

Ingredients For The Salad:

-3 Cups of Water

-1 Cup of Quinoa, Uncooked

-½ tsp. of Salt

-4 Cups of Romaine Lettuce, Thinly Sliced

-1/3 Cup of Apricots, Dried and Cut Into Quarters

-1/3 Cup of Raisins, Golden In Color

-¼ Cup of Pistachios, Dry Roasted and Shelled

-¼ Cup of Green Onions, Finely Sliced

-¼ Cup of Parsley, Fresh and Chopped Finely

-¼ Cup of Cilantro, Fresh and Finely Chopped

-2 Tbsp. of Mint, Fresh and Finely Chopped

-¼ tsp. of Black Pepper, Ground

Ingredients For Dressing:

-½ tsp. of Lime Rind, Finely Grated

-2 Tbsp. of Lime Juice, Fresh

-2 Tbsp. of White Wine, Sweet

-1 Tbsp. of Olive Oil

-½ to 1 tsp. of Jalapeno Pepper, Minced

-¼ tsp. of Salt

-¼ tsp. of Cumin, Ground

-¼ tsp. of Coriander, Ground

-¼ tsp. of Paprika

Directions:

1. To make your salad you will first want to cook your quinoa. To do this place your quinoa into a medium sized saucepan with some water and allow to come to a rolling boil. Once it reaches a boil reduce the heat to a simmer and

allow your quinoa to cook for 15 minutes. Remove from heat and fluff with a fork. Then combine your cooked quinoa with all of your ingredients for your salad and toss lightly to combine all of the ingredients. Set aside.

2. To prepare your dressing for your salad combine all of your ingredients together in a small sized mixing bowl and whisk with a whisk until it is a smooth consistency.

3. To serve, add a generous amount of your quinoa salad to a salad plate and top with some dressing. Serve immediately and enjoy.

Mouthwatering Cajun Style Quinoa Crab Cakes

This recipe is one that you will want to make for nearly any kind of special occasion. This dish will surely impress all of your friends and family and leave them craving more.

Total Prep Time: 50 Minutes

Serves: 4

Ingredients:

-4 Cups of Water, Warm

-1/2 Cup of Quinoa, Uncooked

-1 Sprig of Thyme, Finely Chopped

-1/2 tsp. of Black Pepper, Ground

-1/2 tsp. of Paprika, Ground

-1/4 tsp. of Red Pepper, Ground

-1/4 Cup of Greek Yogurt, Fat Free and Plain In Flavor

-1/4 Cup of Mayonnaise, Canola

-1/4 Cup of Sweet Pickles, Finely Chopped

-1 tsp. of Mustard, Dijon

-8 Ounces of Crab Meat, Shells Removed and Drained

-¼ Cup of Celery, Finely Chopped

-¼ Cup of Red Bell Pepper, Finely Chopped

-¼ Cup of Green Onions, Chopped Finely

-½ tsp. of Salt

-1 Egg White, Large In Size

-2 Tbsp. of Olive Oil, Evenly Divided

Directions:

1. First bring together your first 3 ingredients in a small to medium sized saucepan and stir until all of the ingredients are combined thoroughly. Bring this mixture to a boil. Once it reaches a boil reduce the heat and allow to simmer for the next 15-20 minutes or until there is no liquid left. Remove from heat and fluff your cooked quinoa with a fork. Set aside to allow to cool.

2. Next using a small sized mixing bowl combine your yogurt, ground black pepper,

mustard, red pepper, pickles and paprika until everything is mixed well.

3. Then take your crab meat and place into a medium sized mixing bowl. Mash it slightly. Then add in your yogurt mixture and cooked quinoa and mix with your hands to mix. Then add in your remaining ingredients except for the olive oil and mix again with your hands to combine everything well. Shape the meat into small sized patties and place onto a baking sheet lined with parchment paper. Place the meat into your fridge to set for at least 20 minutes.

4. After 20 minutes remove your crab cakes and set your oven to broiler. Brush the tops of your crab cakes with your olive oil and place into your oven to broil for 5 minutes or until the tops are brown in color. Turn your cakes and brush with some more olive oil. Allow to broil for another 5 minutes or until fully

browned and then remove from oven. Serve whenever you want and thoroughly enjoy.

Red Pepper, Tomato and Squash Alla Gratin

This is another great recipe that you can make for any special occasion. It will please even the pickiest of eaters and will leave them wanting more of this dish.

Total Prep Time: 1 Hour

Serves: 6

Ingredients:

-5 tsp. of Olive Oil, Evenly Divided

-2 Cups of Red Onion, Chopped Finely

-1 ½ Cups of Red Bell Pepper, Finely Chopped

-1 Pound of Yellow Squash, Sliced Into ¼ Inch

Slices

-1 Tbsp. of Garlic, Minced

-½ Cup of Quinoa, Cooked

-½ Cup of Basil, Fresh, Slice Thinly and Evenly Divided

-1 ½ tsp. of Thyme, Fresh and Chopped Coarsely

-¾ tsp. of Salt, Evenly Divided

-½ tsp. of Black Pepper, Ground

-½ Cup of Milk, 2% Reduced Fat

-3 Ounces of Parmesan Cheese, Shredded

-3 Eggs, Large In Size and Beaten Lightly

-Some Cooking Spray

-1 ½ Ounces of French Bread, Fresh and Torn

-1, 12 Ounce Tomato, Beefsteak Variety, Seeded and Cut Into 8 Thin Slices

Directions:

1. Preheat your oven to 375 degrees. While your oven heats up take out a large sized skillet over medium to high heat. Add in half of your oil and add in your onion. Saute for about 3 minutes before adding in your bell pepper. Cook for an additional 2 minutes then add in your garlic and squash to sauté for an additional 5 minutes. Remove from heat and spoon this mixture into a bowl.

2. In this bowl add in your quinoa, thyme, salt, pepper and basil and stir until all of the ingredients are combined thoroughly.

3. In a separate mixing bowl add in your salt, eggs, cheese and milt and stir with a whisk to combine evenly. Add in your veggie mixture and stir again to combine everything. Take out a medium sized baking dish and grease with some cooking spray. Spoon in your milk and veggie mixture into your dish.

4. Using a food processor pulse your French bread until your have coarse bread crumbs. Using your skillet with some olive oil, pour your breadcrumbs into it and cook for about 3 minutes or until the crumbs are lightly toasted.

5. Arrange your tomato slices on your dish and finally top with your toasted breadcrumbs. Place into your oven and bake for 40 minutes or until the top of your dish is lightly browned. Remove from oven and top with some more basil. Serve while still piping hot.

Yummy Red Quinoa Salad

Whenever you wish to spice up your salad dish, this is certainly the recipe you will want to use. Red quinoa helps to make a salad dish much more colorful while adding a unique taste to your salad as well.

Total Prep Time: 45 Minutes

Serves: 4

Ingredients:

-1 Cup of Red Quinoa, Uncooked

-1/3 Cup of Olive Oil

-2 Tbsp. of Vinegar, Red Wine

-1 ½ tsp. of Shallots, Minced Finely

-¼ tsp. of Salt

-¼ tsp. of Black Pepper, Ground

-2 Cups of Tomato, Finely Diced and Seeded

-½ Cup of Cucumber, Finely Diced and Seeded

-3 Tbsp. of Mint, Fresh and Coarsely Chopped

-1 Tbsp. of Oregano, Fresh and Finely Chopped

-1, 15 Ounce Can of Chickpeas, Drained and Rinsed Thoroughly

-2 Ounces of Feta Cheese, Crumbled

-4 Wedges of Lemon, Fresh

Directions:

1. Take your quinoa and cook according to the directions given to you. Once it is fully cooked pour into a bowl and set aside to use for later.

2. While your quinoa begins to cool, combine your olive oil, shallots, Salt and red wine vinegar in a small sized mixing bowl and whisk to stir thoroughly. Allow this mixture to stand for about 20 minutes.

3. Add the rest of your ingredients except for the lemon wedges to your quinoa along with your red vinegar mixture and toss lightly to combine all of the ingredients thoroughly. Spoon a generous helping of the salad into salad bowls and top with your lemon wedges. Serve immediately and enjoy.

Toasted Pine Nuts and Quinoa

This is the perfect side dish that you can make to help compliment any kind of meat based dish that you may be preparing. With its toasted nuttiness flavor, this dish is one that will surely go great with whatever you plan to make for dinner.

Total Prep Time: 30 Minutes

Serves: 4

Ingredients:

-1 Cup of Quinoa, Uncooked

-2 tsp. of Olive Oil, Extra Virgin

-2 Tbsp. of Shallots, Chopped Finely

-1 Tbsp. of Garlic, Minced

-1 ¼ Cups of Chicken Stock, Unsalted

-¼ tsp. of Salt

-¼ Cup of Pine Nuts, Fresh

-1 Tbsp. of Olive Oil, Extra Virgin

-¼ Cup of Parsley, Fresh and Chopped Finely

-2 Tbsp. of Chives, Fresh and Chopped Finely

-¼ tsp. of Black Pepper, Ground

Directions:

1. The first thing you will need to do is rinse and drain your quinoa thoroughly. Once that is done take out a medium sized saucepan and heat it up over medium heat. Add in your extra virgin olive oil and saute your shallots for about 1 minute or until the shallots become tender. Next add in your garlic and cook for an additional minute, making sure to stir as frequently as possible.

2. Then add in your quinoa and cook for another 2 minutes, stirring as frequently as possible. Then add in your chicken stock and

salt and stir to combine all of the ingredient. Bring this mixture to a boil and then reduce the heat to a simmer. Cover with a lid and allow your mixture to simmer for 15 minutes or until all of the liquid has been absorbed. Remove from heat and fluff your tender quinoa with a fork. Set aside.

3. Take out a small sized saucepan and toss in your pine nuts. Allow to cook for 3 minutes or until the nuts are lightly browned. Combine with your cooked quinoa and add in your chives, pepper, olive oil and chopped parsley. Toss lightly to combine and serve immediately.

Fresh Baked Tomatoes With Quinoa and Green Chilies

If you are a fan of stuffed tomatoes, then you are going to love this dish. This recipe includes stuffed tomatoes that are packed full of healthy quinoa and sweet corn. It is covered with melted cheese which will surely leave your guests mouths watering.

Total Prep Time: 1 Hour and 5 Minutes

Serves: 6

Ingredients:

-2 Poblano Chilies, Finely Chopped

-2 Cups of Corn Kernels, Fresh

-1 Cup of Onion, Chopped Finely

-1 Tbsp. of Oregano, Fresh and Chopped Finely

-1 Tbsp. of Olive Oil

-1 Tbsp. of Lime Juice, Fresh

-1 tsp. of Salt, Evenly Divided

-¾ tsp. of Cumin, Ground

-¼ tsp. of Black Pepper, Ground and Fresh

-6 Tomatoes, Ripe

-1 Cup of Quinoa, Uncooked

-¼ Cup of Water

-4 Ounces of Colby Jack Cheese, Shredded

Directions:

1. Preheat your oven to broiler. While this heats up prepare your chilies by slicing them in half lengthwise and clean out the insides. Place your chilies onto a baking sheet and broil for at least 8 minutes or until the chilies are fully blackened. Remove from heat and chop your chilies finely.

2. Add in your onions and corn to your baking pan and place into your oven to broil to cook for 10 minutes, making sure to stir at least twice. Once done add to your chopped up chilies. Add in your lime juice, black pepper, oregano, salt and cumin and toss lightly to

combine thoroughly. Set aside.

3. Next cut the tops of your tomatoes and set the tops aside. Being as careful as you can scoop out your tomato pulp from the insides of your tomatoes. Sprinkle your tomatoes with some salt and allow to stand for at least 30 minutes.

4. Prepare your quinoa according to the directions on the package and once your quinoa is fully cooked, add it to your corn mixture. Toss the ingredients together to combine.

5. Preheat your oven to 350 degrees. While it heats up scoop about ¾ cup of your corn mixture into each of your tomatoes. Sprinkle your cheese on top of each tomato and place into your oven to bake.

6. Bake your tomatoes for 15 minutes. After 15 minutes remove from your oven and set your oven to broil. Broil your tomatoes for an

additional 12 minutes or until the cheese fully melts on top. Remove from oven and serve as soon as possible.

Spicy Shrimp Grilled With Quinoa

If you are looking for a dish that packs one hell of a punch, this is the perfect dish for you. This recipe makes a dish that packs a triple punch and that is incredibly high in healthy protein.

Total Prep Time: 50 Minutes

Serves: 4

Ingredients:

-¼ Cup of Lime Juice, Fresh and Evenly Divided

-10 tsp. of Olive Oil, Evenly Divided

-2 tsp. of Chili Powder

-1 tsp. of Cumin, Ground and Evenly Divided

-¼ tsp. of Black Pepper

-¼ tsp. of Hot Sauce, Your Favorite Kind

-1/8 tsp. of Paprika, Smoked and Spanish Style

-4 Cloves of Garlic, Finely Chopped and Evenly Divided

-24 Pieces of Shrimp, Large in Size, Deveined and Peeled

-¾ Cup of Quinoa, Uncooked

-½ Cup of Onion, Finely Chopped

-1 Cup of Water, Warm

-½ tsp. of Salt, Evenly Divided

-½ tsp. of Honey

-1 Cup of Tomatoes, Cherry and Evenly Divided

-½ Cup of Chickpeas, Canned, Rinsed and

Drained

-½ Cup of Avocado, Peeled and Finely Diced

-1 Ounce of Feta Cheese, Crumbled

-Some Cooking Spray

-¼ Cup of Cilantro, Fresh and Finely Chopped

Directions:

1. Prepare a grill by preheating to high heat. While it heats up take out a small sized mixing bowl and combine your 2 cloves of garlic, olive oil, cumin, chili powder, hot sauce, black pepper and paprika and stir thoroughly to combine evenly. Add your shrimp to this mixture by tossing it lightly and place into your fridge to marinate for the next 30 minutes.

2. While your shrimp marinated you will then need to prepare your quinoa. To do this heat up 1 Tbsp. of olive oil in a medium sized saucepan over medium to high heat. Sauté your onions

for 3 minutes or until they are tender. Then add in your quinoa and garlic and cook for another 2 minutes, making sure to stir constantly. Then add in your water and bring to a rolling boil. Reduce the heat to a simmer and allow your quinoa mixture to simmer for 15 minutes or until all of the liquid has been absorbed. Fluff your quinoa with a fork and then add in your fresh lime juice, cumin, salt, olive oil and honey. Stir until thoroughly mixed.

3. Next add in your chickpeas, cheese, tomatoes and avocado to your mixture and toss to combine all of the ingredients.

4. Remove your shrimp from the bowl of marinade and season with a dash of salt. Pierce your shrimp onto thin skewers and place onto grill. Grill your shrimp for at least 2 minutes on each side or until the shrimp is fully cook. Remove from grill.

5. Divide up your quinoa mixture onto a few plate and top with your fully cooked shrimp. Serve immediately.

Nutritious Breakfast Style Quinoa

Like most grains available today, quinoa is one of those that is surprisingly filling. If this does not fill you up, do not hesitate to serve this up with a side of eggs to make a delicious and filling breakfast dish.

Total Prep Time: 35 Minutes

Serves: 4

Ingredients:

-½ Cup of Quinoa, Uncooked

-2 Tbsp. of Water, Warm

-¾ Cup of Coconut Milk, Light

-1 Tbsp. of Brown Sugar, Light

-1/8 tsp. of Salt

-1 Cup of Strawberries, Sliced Thinly

-¼ Cup of Coconut, Unsweetened and Flaked

-1 Cup of Bananas, Sliced Thinly

Directions:

1. Preheat your oven to 400 degrees. While it heats up prepare your quinoa by placing it into a small saucepan with your coconut milk, brown sugar, water and salt and bring the mixture to a rolling boil. Reduce the heat and allow to simmer until all of the liquid has been absorbed. This should take about 15 to 20 minutes.

2. As your quinoa cooks take out a baking sheet and layer your flaked coconut into the bottom of the sheet. Bake this for 5 minutes or until the coconut flakes turn golden brown in color.

3. Pour your quinoa into small sized bowl and top with your sliced strawberries and bananas. Finish off by topping it with your toasted coconut flakes. Serve while the dish is still warm and enjoy.

Fast Quinoa Meatballs

This recipe is an excellent one to make especially if you are on a low sodium diet. Serve this with a dish of pasta or eat as a snack by itself.

Total Prep Time: 40 Minutes

Serves: 6

Ingredients:

-½ Cup of Quinoa, Wash and Uncooked

-1 Pound of Pork, Ground

-½ Cup of Shallots, Finely Diced

-4 Cloves of Garlic, Smashed

-2 Eggs, Large

-½ tsp. of Black Pepper, Ground

-½ tsp. of Cayenne Pepper, Ground

-½ tsp. of Paprika, Ground

-½ tsp. of Oregano, Dried

-½ tsp. of Parsley, Dried

-¼ tsp. of Cinnamon, Ground

Directions:

1. Preheat your oven to 450 degrees. While it heats up line a baking sheet with some parchment paper and set aside.

2. Prepare your quinoa according to the directions listed on the package. Once your quinoa is fully cooked remove from heat and allow to cool for a couple of minutes.

3. As your quinoa cools add the rest of your ingredients into a medium sized mixing bowl. Using your hands mix up all of the ingredients together until they are thoroughly combined.

4. Shape your mixture into evenly sized balls and place them evenly onto your baking sheet. Place this into your oven and bake for the next 12 to 15 minutes or until they are golden brown in color. Remove from your oven and serve with a side of pasta or serve by themselves immediately.

Sesame Quinoa

The almonds that you will use in this recipe will help you to balance out this dish nicely. The red quinoa you use will give this dish a unique red color as well as savory taste.

Total Prep Time: 25 Minutes

Serves: 4

Ingredients:

-1 2/3 Cups of Water, Warm

-1 Cup of Red Quinoa, Uncooked

-2 Tbsp. of Lemon Juice, Fresh

-¼ Cup of Almonds, Toasted and Sliced Thinly

-2 tsp. of Olive Oil

-2 tsp. of Sesame Oil, Dark in Color

-¼ tsp. of Salt

-3 Green Onion, Sliced Thinly

Directions:

1. To prepare your red quinoa you will want to bring your water and quinoa to a rolling boil in a medium sized saucepan. Cover with a lid and reduce the heat to a simmer. Allow your quinoa to cook for the next 15 to 20 minutes or until

the water has been fully absorbed. Remove from heat and fluff your cooked red quinoa with a fork. Stir in your sliced onions, toasted almonds, salt, sesame oil and olive oil. Stir to thoroughly combine.

2. Add in your lemon juice and stir to combine. Serve into a bowl and enjoy immediately.

Spicy Quinoa and Bean Salad

With this dish you can enjoy a great tasting salad that has a bit of a kick to it. Feel free to be as creative with your ingredients as possible to make this dish unique in your household.

Total Prep Time: 5 Minutes

Serves: 6

Ingredients:

-1 tsp. of Orange Rind, Grated

-½ tsp. of Cumin, Ground

-¾ tsp. of Cocoa, Unsweetened

-½ tsp. of Cinnamon, Ground

-2 Tbsp. of Orange Juice, Fresh

-1 ½ Tbsp. of Vinegar, Red Wine

-1 Tbsp. of Adobo Sauce

-2 Tbsp. of Olive Oil

-3 Cups of Quinoa, Fully Cooked and Cooled

-½ Cup of Pumpkinseed Kernels, Unsalted and Toasted

-¼ Cup of Cilantro, Fresh and Finely Chopped

-½ tsp. of Salt

-2 Green Onions, Sliced Thinly

-1 Jalapeno Pepper, Fresh and Thinly Sliced

-1, 15 Ounce Can of Black Beans, Rinsed and Drained Beforehand

-4 Cups of Baby Spinach, Whole Leaves

Directions:

1. To prepare combine your first 7 ingredients in a small sized bowl. Stir to evenly combine and then gradually add in your olive oil, making sure to stir the entire time.

2. Then combine your next 6 ingredients as well as your cooked quinoa in a large sized mixing bowl. Toss gently to mix well and add your vinaigrette into it. Toss again to coat everything evenly.

3. Next add in your whole baby spinach leaves and toss again to combine everything together. Serve immediately and enjoy.

Conclusion

After reading this eBook and going through the various recipes listed in here, I hope that you are inspired to create dishes centered around this healthy grain. You will learn after making your first few quinoa based recipes that quinoa is pretty easy to prepare and tastes even better once it is done.

The quinoa recipes that you can find both in books and online are virtually endless. With many people turning over to include this grain into their daily diet, more people are becoming inspired to create great tasting dishes centered around this grain.

There are many reasons why you should include quinoa in your daily diet and with this eBook I hope that I have helped you take your first step into the world of quinoa cooking and on the path to a healthier lifestyle.

About Us

The Thought Flame is committed to add value to its customers through various books, online courses and other resources. You can learn more about us and our books at www.thethoughtflame.com.

Don't forget to check out our amazing **online video courses** at www.thethoughtflame.com/courses/ to take your knowledge to another level.

To check out our **extraordinary collection of diet/cookbooks**, visit http://www.thethoughtflame.com/category/non-fictional/cookbooks/ .

As a part of our valued relationship with our customers, we keep providing you free promotional books, courses and other stuff on subscribing with us on our site. We have a strict anti-spam policy and assure you no spam mails will be sent to your mailbox.

To subscribe with us, visit www.thethoughtflame.com.

Like our work and would like to say thanks? Buy us a cup of coffee at www.thethoughtflame.com/coffee/

Author

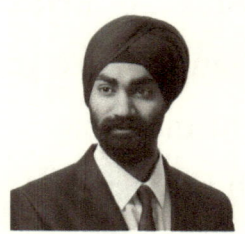

Amarpreet Singh is an avid learner and his passion for education has made him travel, work and study all across the world. He holds three masters degrees, including MBA, from top universities in Asia.

He is author of dozens of books, many of which are Amazon's bestseller, varying in various topics and categories. He also teaches many online courses having thousands of students across the world.

He has a keen interest in international affairs, economics, global poverty and politics, financial markets and entrepreneurship, and strives to be part of a community that shares the same passion.

He has worked as consultant with organizations like Airbus and The World Bank. He loves travelling and learning about new cultures, and has been fortunate to live/work/travel/study in countries like India, China, Korea, US, South Africa, Japan, Philippines, Singapore, Canada etc., and learn about the culture and lifestyle in each of them. To check out more of his work, visit www.thethoughtflame.com

www.ingramcontent.com/pod-product-compliance
Lightning Source LLC
Chambersburg PA
CBHW050421290526
45786CB00003B/1352